Published By Robert Corbin

@ Natalie Kappen

Clean Diet: The Beginner-friendly Guide to Clean

Eating Diet for Great Health and Clean Living

All Right RESERVED

ISBN 978-1-7385954-0-2

TABLE OF CONTENTS

Healthy Cabbage Soup 1

Fall Seasoned Soup... 3

Banana Hemp Shake 5

Raspberry Smoothie Bowl 6

Clean Eating Cobb Salad 8

Skinny Slow Cooker – Balsamic Chicken.......................... 10

Air Fryer French Toast Soldiers 12

Baked Chicken With Peppers 14

Chicken And Vegetable Kebabs With Orzo 17

Classic Deviled Eggs... 20

Greek Meatball Mezze Bowls.. 22

Squash & Red Lentil Curry... 25

Pea Salad With Corn.. 28

Potatoes With Peas And Gravy 30

Pesto And Egg Breakfast Bake... 32

Heartwarming Cinnamon And Cherry Oats................... 34

Chicken Kiev With A Cucumber And Spring Onion Salad 36

Slow-Cooked Chicken Thighs With Gravy 41

Guilt-Free Beef Kebabs 46

Blackened Chicken With Avocado 48

Chia Pudding Almond Yogurt Parfait With Warm Cranberries 50

Spice Porridge With Oranges And Pears 52

Totally Awesome Tomato, Cucumber & Over-The-Top Orange Soup 54

Spicy Chunky Chicken Tangy Tomato Soup 57

Thai Style Tomato Soup 60

Traditional Mexican Bean Salad 62

Avocado Almond Smoothie Bowl 64

Strawberry Cream Shake 66

Quinoa Breakfast Cereal 68

Spinach & Bean Burrito Wrap 70

Chicken Tostadas 72

Instant Pot Stir Fry 74

Coffee-Rubbed Steak With Brussels Sprouts Salad 77

Crispy Salmon Salad With Roasted Butternut Squash ... 80

Vegetarian Recipes Goes Thus; White Beans With Roasted Red Pepper And Pesto 83

Black Lentil And Couscous Salad 87

Schnitzel With Vegetables 89

Risotto With Peas 91

Refrigerator Berry Citrus Breakfast Pudding 93

Spicy Morning Breakfast Cocktail 95

Avocado Toast With Radish Ceviche 97

Crab With Mango And Avocado Salad 99

Grilled Vegetable Wraps With Salsa And Guacamole .. 101

Breakfast: Banana Blueberry Pancakes 105

Chicken With Lemon Garlic Sauce 107

Acai Blackberry Smoothie Bowl 109

Crazy Carrot, Potatoes & Celery Soup 111

Crazy Cauliflower & Bacon Soup 115

Chunky Chicken & Vegetable Soup 118

Fresh Spinach And Strawberry Salad 122

Grilled Balsamic Veggie Salad 124

Millet With Fruit And Walnuts 126

Peanut Butter Green Smoothie..................................... 128

Golden Turmeric Smoothie 129

Quinoa Salad With Seasonal Vegetables....................... 131

Honey Glazed Salmon With Lemon.............................. 135

Chicken Breast With Tomatoes 137

One Pot Quinoa, Chicken And Broccoli 140

Ground Chicken Tacos... 143

Eggs Benedict On Greens With Yogurt Hollandaise Sauce 146

Cinnamon And Maple Sweet Potato Waffles............... 149

Quick Avocado Chocolate Mousse................................ 151

Healthy Cabbage Soup

Ingredients:

- 3 cups of water, warm
- 1 head of cabbage, shredded
- 2 tbsp. Of tomato paste, fresh
- ½ of a lemon, juiced
- Dash of salt and pepper for taste
- 1 tbsp. Of cilantro, chopped finely
- 1 tsp. Of thyme, dried
- 2 tbsp. Of olive oil
- 1 red bell pepper, cored and sliced finely
- 1 green bell pepper, cored and sliced finely
- 1 onion, medium in size and chopped finely

Directions:

1. Using a large sized saucepan, heat up your olive oil over medium to high heat.
2. Add in your onion and sauté it for the next 2 to 3 minutes.
3. Next add in your peppers and cabbage and allow to cook for the next 5 minutes.
4. After 5 minutes add in your water and tomato paste. Stir until combined evenly.
5. Then add in your dash of salt and pepper for taste and stir again.
6. Allow the soup to cook over medium heat for the next 20 to 30 minutes.
7. After this time add in the rest of your INGREDIENTS:and stir to combine evenly.
8. Serve into bowls and enjoy immediately.

Fall Seasoned Soup

Ingredients:

- 1 pinch of cinnamon powder, ground

- 1 pinch of cardamom, ground

- 1 tomato, ripe and finely chopped

- 3 cups of vegetable stock, low in sodium

- ¼ tsp. Of anise seeds

- 1 red bell pepper, cored and chopped finely

- 1 cup of water, warm

- Dash of salt and pepper for taste

- ¼ cup of walnuts, chopped and to be used for serving

- 2 tbsp. Of olive oil

- 1 clove of garlic, chopped finely
- 1 onion, medium in size and finely chopped
- 4 cups of butternut squash, chopped into cubes

Directions:

1. Using a large soup pot, heat up your olive oil over medium heat.
2. Add in your onion and garlic and sauté for the next 2 minutes or until fragrant.
3. Then stir in the rest of your INGREDIENTS:except for the chopped walnuts until evenly combined.
4. Allow to cook for the next 20 to 30 minutes.
5. Remove from heat and pour into a blender to puree until it reaches the right consistency.
6. Serve and top with chopped walnuts. Enjoy.

Banana Hemp Shake

Ingredients:

- 2 bananas, very ripe, frozen
- ¼ cup PB2
- 2 tbsp hemp protein powder or any protein powder of your choice
- 2 Medjool dates, large, pitted & soaked for half an hour
- 1 cup hemp milk

Directions:
1. Put everything together, preferably in the order mentioned above in a high-powered mixer or food processor; process on high settings until smooth.
2. Serve chilled.

Raspberry Smoothie Bowl

Ingredients:

For the Raspberry Smoothie

- 1 packet of Vega Vanilla Protein Powder
- 1 cup almond milk
- 2 tbsp. water plus 2 tbsp. chia seeds
- 1 cup raspberries, frozen
- 1 banana, small, frozen

For toppings

- 1/4 cup Vanilla Almond flavor granola
- Cacao nibs
- A few raspberries, fresh

Directions:

1. Soak the chia seeds in water until thick & gelatinous, for 10 minutes.
2. Transfer the soaked chia seeds to a blender, along with all of the remaining smoothie Ingredients:; blend on high settings until smooth.
3. Pour the mixture into a large bowl & top it with the granola, cacao nibs, & fresh raspberries.
4. Serve with a large spoon. Enjoy.

Clean Eating Cobb Salad

Ingredients:

Salad

- 1 split chicken breast, cooked, skin removed and cubed

- 2 vine-ripe tomatoes, chopped

- 2 hard-boiled eggs, peeled and sliced

- 6 cups chopped romaine heart lettuce

- 2 ripe avocados, seeded and peeled, slice into 1" pieces

Dressing

- 1 teaspoon honey or maple syrup

- Kosher or sea salt to taste

- 1/8 teaspoon black pepper

- 1/4 cup red-wine vinegar

- 1/2 cup extra-virgin olive oil

Directions:
1. Combine salad INGREDIENTS:in a large bowl.
2. Combine dressing INGREDIENTS:and drizzle over salad.

Skinny Slow Cooker – Balsamic Chicken

Ingredients:

- 1/2 cup of balsamic vinegar
- 1 tablespoon of olive oil
- 1 teaspoon of dried oregano
- 1 teaspoon of dried basil
- 1 teaspoon of dried rosemary
- 1/2 teaspoon of thyme
- 4-6 boneless chicken breasts (40 ounces)
- 2 14.5 oz of can diced tomatoes
- 1 medium-sized onion thinly sliced (not chopped)
- 4 garlic cloves

- Black pepper and salt

Directions:
1. Pour the olive oil on the lower part of a moderate cooker, add chicken bosoms, salt, and pepper each bosom, put cut onion on top of chicken at that point put in all the dried spices and garlic cloves.
2. Pour in vinegar and top with tomatoes.
3. Cook on high for 4 hours, serve over holy messenger hair pasta.

Air Fryer French Toast Soldiers

Ingredients:

- ¼ Cup whole milk
- ¼ cup brown sugar
- 1 tbsp honey
- 1 tsp cinnamon
- Pinch of nutmeg
- Philips airfryer
- 4 slices wholemeal bread
- 2 large eggs
- Pinch of icing sugar

Directions:

1. Chop up your slices of bread into soldiers. Each slice should make 4 soldiers.
2. Place the rest of your Ingredients: (apart from the icing sugar) into a mixing bowl and mix well.
3. Dip each soldier into the mixture so that it is well coated and then place it into the Air Fryer.
4. When you're done you will have 16 soldiers and then should all be nice and wet from the mixture.
5. Place on 160c for 10 minutes or until they are nice and crispy like toast and are no longer wet.
6. Halfway through cooking turn them over so that both sides of the soldiers have a good chance to be evenly cooked.
7. Serve with a sprinkle of icing sugar and some fresh berries.

Baked Chicken With Peppers

Ingredients:

- 1 medium onion, finely chopped

- 10 brown mushrooms or 2 portobellos, chopped

- 2 large bell peppers, chopped

- 1 tbsp coconut or avocado oil

- 1 cup hard cheese like mozzarella or marble, shredded

- 3 lbs chicken breasts or thighs, boneless & skinless

- 1 large garlic clove, grated

- 1/2 tsp himalayan pink salt

- Ground black pepper, to taste

Directions:

1. Preheat oven to 425 degrees. Rinse chicken and if using breasts cut in half lengthwise. In a large baking dish, add chicken, garlic, salt and pepper. Mix well to coat evenly and spread in a single layer. Cover and bake for 20-25 minutes. Chicken is cooked when pale and surrounded by clear juices.
2. In the meanwhile, preheat large ceramic non-stick skillet on low-medium heat and swirl oil to coat. Add onion and saute for a few minutes, stirring occasionally.
3. Add mushrooms and saute for a few more minutes, stirring occasionally. Add bell peppers and saute for 5 more minutes, stirring.
4. Remove chicken from the oven and turn broiler on High. Separate chicken a bit from each other and top each piece with

vegetables (sprinkle around too) and top with cheese.
5. Broil for 5 minutes or until cheese is melted.
6. Serve hot with rice, quinoa or veggies.

Chicken And Vegetable Kebabs With Orzo

Ingredients:

- 1/2 teaspoon black pepper, divided
- 3 6 3 (6-oz.) sweet potatoes
- 1 yellow bell pepper, cut into 1 1/2-inch pieces
- 2 tablespoons olive oils, divided
- 1 bunch scallions
- 2 cups cooked whole-wheat orzo
- 1/4 cup sour cream
- 1 pound boneless, skinless chicken breast, cut into 1-inch pieces
- 3 tablespoons fresh lime juice, divided

- 1 tablespoon minced chipotle chiles in adobo sauce plus 1/2 tbs adobo sauce

- 1 teaspoon kosher salt , divided

Directions:
1. Toss chicken with 1 tablespoon lime juice, chipotle chiles, adobo sauce, 1/2 teaspoon salt, and 1/4 teaspoon pepper. Let stand 10 minutes. Thread chicken onto 3 (12-inch) metal skewers.
2. Pierce potatoes with a fork. Wrap with damp paper towels, and microwave at high until slightly tender, about 3 minutes.
3. Cut into 1/2-inch rounds. Thread sweet potatoes and bell pepper alternately onto 2 (12-inch) metal skewers.
4. Whisk together 1 tablespoon lime juice, 1 tablespoon oil, 1/4 teaspoon salt, and remaining 1/4 teaspoon pepper. Brush half of dressing on vegetables.

5. Preheat grill to high (450°F to 550°F). Place chicken on oiled grates; grill, uncovered, until cooked through, 6 to 8 minutes.
6. Grill vegetables, uncovered, brushing with half of remaining dressing, until tender, 4 to 6 minutes.
7. Brush scallions with remaining dressing; grill, uncovered, until charred, 2 to 3 minutes.
8. Chop scallions; toss with orzo, remaining 1 tablespoon oil, and remaining 1/4 teaspoon salt.
9. Combine sour cream and remaining 1 tablespoon lime juice. Serve with skewers.

Classic Deviled Eggs

Ingredients:

- 1 teaspoon apple cider vinegar
- 3/8 teaspoon kosher salt
- 1/8 teaspoon black pepper
- 1/8 teaspoon smoked paprika
- 6 large eggs
- 1/4 cup canola mayonnaise
- 1 teaspoon dijon mustard

Directions:

1. Fill a medium saucepan with 1-inch of water; fit with a steamer basket and bring to a boil over high heat.
2. Add eggs, cover, and steam until hard-cooked, about 13 minutes.

3. Transfer eggs to an ice bath and let sit until chilled, about 6 minutes.
4. Peel. Discard shells.
5. Halve eggs. Scoop yolks into a medium bowl.
6. Add mayo, mustard, vinegar, salt, and pepper; mix until smooth. Scoop mixture into a zip-top bag and cut off corner.
7. Pipe yolk mixture evenly between whites. Sprinkle evenly with paprika. Serve immediately.

Greek Meatball Mezze Bowls

Ingredients:

- ½ teaspoon garlic powder

- ½ teaspoon dried oregano

- ⅜ teaspoon salt, divided

- ⅜ teaspoon ground pepper, divided

- 2 cups cooked quinoa, cooled (see Associated Recipes)

- 2 tablespoons lemon juice

- 1 tablespoon olive oil

- 1 cup frozen chopped spinach, thawed

- 1 pound 93%-lean ground turkey

- ½ cup crumbled feta cheese

- ½ cup chopped parsley
- 3 tablespoons chopped mint
- 2 cups sliced cucumber
- 1 pint cherry tomatoes
- ¼ cup tzatziki

Directions:
1. Squeeze excess moisture from spinach.
2. Combine the spinach with turkey, feta, garlic powder, oregano, 1/8 teaspoon salt and 1/8 teaspoon pepper in a medium bowl; mix well.
3. Form the mixture into 12 meatballs. Heat a large nonstick skillet over medium heat.
4. Coat with cooking spray. Working in batches if necessary, add the meatballs to the pan and cook until browned on all sides and no longer pink in the center, about 10 to 12 minutes.

5. (An instant-read thermometer inserted in the center should register 165 degrees F.) Set the meatballs aside to cool.
6. Combine quinoa, lemon juice, oil, parsley, mint and the remaining 1/4 teaspoon each salt and pepper in a medium bowl.
7. Divide among 4 single-serving lidded containers.
8. Top each with 3 meatballs, 1/2 cup cucumbers and 1/2 cup cherry tomatoes.
9. Seal the containers and refrigerate for up to 4 days. Divide tzatziki among 4 small containers and refrigerate.

Before serving, transfer the meatballs to a microwave-safe container and heat until steaming. Return to the original container and serve with tzatziki.

Squash & Red Lentil Curry

Ingredients:

- 1 20-ounce package cubed peeled butternut squash (see Tip)
- 1 cup red lentils
- 1 cup chopped fresh tomato or one 15-ounce can diced tomatoes, drained
- 1 ½ teaspoons salt
- 4 cups water
- 1 14-ounce can lite coconut milk
- 5 lime wedges
- Chopped fresh cilantro for garnish
- 2 tablespoons canola oil

- 1 ½ cups diced onion
- 2 cloves garlic, minced
- 1 tablespoon minced fresh ginger
- 2 teaspoons curry powder or garam masala

Directions:

1. Heat oil in a large pot over medium-high heat. Add onion, garlic, ginger and curry powder (or garam masala); cook, stirring often, until the onion is starting to soften, 2 to 3 minutes.
2. Add squash, lentils, tomato and salt; cook, stirring, for 1 minute. Add water.
3. Cover and bring to a boil over high heat.
4. Reduce heat to maintain a lively simmer; cook, covered, stirring occasionally, until the squash is tender and the lentils are mostly broken down, about 20 minutes.

5. Stir in coconut milk and simmer until heated through, about 1 minute.
6. Serve with lime wedges and cilantro, if desired. Tips
7. Precut butternut s quash is usually sold in a 20-ounce package of large cubes (5 cups of 1- to 2-inch pieces) or in a package of large cubes (5 cups of 1- to 2-inch pieces) or in a inch pieces).
8. If you can only find the smaller cubes for this recipe, you'll need to buy two 16-ounce packages to have 5 total cups of squash and reduce the roasting time by 5 to 10 minutes.
9. Or, you can prep your own cubes of squash from a whole, peeled and seeded butternut squash.

Pea Salad With Corn

Ingredients:

- 1 bunch green onions

- 150g (5.30 oz.) green peas

- 150g (5.30 oz.) corn

- 100g (5.50 oz.) diet yoghurt

- 50g (1.76 oz.) bacon

- 1 tsp. seasoning Kari

- 1 apple, peel and finely cut into cubes

- 1 tsp. lemon juice

- Salt and black pepper to taste

Directions:

1. Cut apple into cubes and drizzle with lemon juice.
2. Finely chop the chives and mix with peas, corn and apples.
3. Add yogurt curry, salt and pepper.
4. Chop bacon and add to the salad along with the sauce.

Potatoes With Peas And Gravy

Ingredients:

- 1 tsp. butter

- 100 ml broth

- 2 tbsp. sour cream

- 2 tablespoons chervil leaves

- 2 large potatoes

- 1 onion

- 200 g (7oz.) green peas

- Salt

Directions:

1. Boil the potatoes in their skins.
2. Chop onions and fry in butter with 150g (5.30 oz.) of green peas.

3. Pour the broth and simmer for 10 minutes.
4. Add 1 tablespoon sour cream add finely chopped chervil and done using a mixer.
5. Add the remaining sauce, peas.
6. Cut potatoes, pour the sauce and the remaining sour cream.

Pesto And Egg Breakfast Bake

Ingredients:

- 2 cloves garlic, crushed and minced
- 1 tablespoon olive oil
- 6 eggs, beaten
- ½ cup milk
- ½ teaspoon thyme
- 1 teaspoon black pepper
- 1 tomato, sliced
- ½ cup fresh basil, chopped
- ¼ cup fresh parsley, chopped
- 2 cups fresh spinach, chopped
- ¼ cup fresh grated parmesan cheese

- ½ cup walnuts, chopped

- Additional fresh basil for garnish, if desired.

Directions:
1. Preheat oven to 375°F/191°C.
2. In a blender or food processor, combine the basil, parsley, spinach, parmesan cheese, walnuts, garlic, and olive oil. Pulse until mixture is smooth.
3. Add the eggs, milk, thyme, and pepper. Blend just until mixed.
4. Lightly oil four 10-ounce ramekins.
5. Pour equal amounts of the mixture into the four ramekins. Top each with a slice of tomato.
6. Place in the oven, and bake for approximately 30 minutes or until set in the middle.
7. Garnish with fresh basil, if desired.

Heartwarming Cinnamon And Cherry Oats

Ingredients:

- ¼ cup local honey
- 1 teaspoon pure vanilla extract
- 1 ¼ cups milk
- 1 egg, beaten
- 2 teaspoons fresh grated ginger
- 1 tablespoon cinnamon
- 2 cups old fashioned rolled oats
- ½ cup ground flax meal
- 1 ½ cup raw almonds, chopped
- 2 cups fresh cherries, pitted and chopped

Directions:

1. Preheat the oven to 350°F/177°C.
2. In a bowl, combine the oats, flax meal, almonds, and cherries. Mix gently.
3. Add the honey and vanilla extract. Mix to coat evenly.
4. Make a well in the center of the mixture, and add in the milk and egg.
5. Slowly incorporate the milk and egg into the rest of the mixture until well mixed.
6. Season with fresh ginger and cinnamon.
7. Transfer to a lightly oiled, 9x9 baking dish. Place in the oven, and bake 25-30 minutes, or until all liquid has been absorbed.

Chicken Kiev With A Cucumber And Spring Onion Salad

Ingredients:

- 50g/1¾oz Cheddar, grated
- salt and freshly ground black pepper
- 2 free-range eggs, beaten
- 3 tbsp plain flour
- 3 tbsp golden breadcrumbs
- sunflower oil, for deep-frying
- 4 chicken breasts, preferably free-range, skin removed
- 150g/5½oz butter, at room temperature
- bunch fresh parsley, finely chopped
- 3 garlic cloves, crushed

- 2 spring onions, finely chopped

For the salad

- large pinch paprika
- salt and freshly ground black pepper
- 2 free-range eggs, hardboiled, peeled, sliced
- 2 cucumbers, peeled, core removed
- 2 spring onions, chopped
- 50g/1¾oz soured cream
- 1 tbsp mayonnaise

Directions:

1. For the kievs, slit each chicken breast down its longer side, almost cutting through to the other side (the breast should open out like a book). Place the opened chicken breast between two pieces of clingfilm and flatten

with a rolling pin. Set aside. Repeat with the remaining three chicken breasts.
2. Mix the butter, parsley, garlic, spring onions and grated cheese in a bowl. Divide this stuffing into four and form each portion into a sausage shape. Set aside.
3. Pour the beaten eggs into a bowl and spread the flour and breadcrumbs onto separate plates.
4. Meanwhile, for the salad, peel the cucumbers into thin ribbons using a vegetable peeler and mix with the spring onions, soured cream, mayonnaise and paprika. Season to taste with salt and freshly ground black pepper. Garnish with the slices of hard-boiled egg. Set the salad aside until ready to serve.
5. Lay a chicken breast flat on a chopping board, season with salt and freshly ground black pepper, and place a portion of stuffing in the middle.

6. Roll the chicken very tightly around the stuffing and then dip in the flour to coat the chicken evenly. Dip into the beaten egg, and then roll in the breadcrumbs. Repeat with the remaining chicken breasts and stuffing.
7. Heat the oil in a deep heavy-based frying pan until a breadcrumb sizzles and turns light golden when dropped into it. Alternatively, use an electric deep-fat fryer heated to 160C/325F. (CAUTION: Hot oil can be dangerous. Do not leave unattended.) NB: it's important that the oil temperature isn't too hot or the outside of the chicken will burn before the inside is cooked.
8. Cook the chicken for about 15 minutes until the coating is golden and crispy and the chicken is cooked through (test the chicken by removing to a plate and piercing with a skewer – the juices will run clear when the chicken is cooked).

9. Remove the chicken from the pan with a slotted spoon and set aside to drain on kitchen paper.
10. Serve the chicken kievs with the cucumber salad alongside.

Slow-Cooked Chicken Thighs With Gravy

Ingredients:

For the chicken gravy

- 2 kombu leaves, rinsed in cold water

- 1 fresh sage leaf

- 1 fresh thyme sprig

- 1 unwaxed lemon, pared zest only

- 500g/1lb 2oz chicken wings

- 1 carrot, peeled and roughly chopped

- 1 onion, roughly chopped

- 1 stick celery, roughly chopped

- ½ leek, roughly chopped

- 4 garlic cloves, roughly chopped

- 1 tbsp tomato purée
- 125ml/4fl oz dry white wine
- 1 Parmesan rind
- 500ml/18fl oz dark chicken stock
- 250ml/9fl oz veal stock

For the chicken thighs

- 1 thyme sprig
- 1 lemon
- 4 boneless chicken thighs
- 100g/3½oz fine sea salt
- 1 bay leaf

For the swede purée

- 1 large swede, peeled and diced

- 200g/7oz butter

- salt and freshly ground black pepper

Directions:

1. To make the gravy, preheat the oven to 220C/200C Fan/Gas 7. Put the chicken wings in a large roasting tray and roast for 30 minutes, or until golden brown.
2. Transfer the chicken to a plate and set aside. Add the vegetables and garlic to the roasting tray and toss in the chicken fat. Roast for 40 minutes, or until golden and caramelised. Put the tray over a high heat and add the tomato purée. Deglaze the pan with the wine, add the Parmesan rind and allow to bubble. Return the chicken wings to the tray and pour in both stocks. Bring to a simmer and cook until reduced.
3. Meanwhile, for the chicken thighs, put 1 litre/1¾ pints water in a large pan and add the

salt. Bring to the boil then remove from the heat. Add the herbs and lemon and allow to cool. Once fridge cold, put the chicken thighs in the brine and leave in the fridge for 1 hour.

4. Remove the chicken thighs from the brine and rinse, then put them in a sous vide bag. Cook them in water bath at 62C for 4 hours.

5. Strain the gravy from the chicken wings into a clean pan and place over a medium heat. Discard the wings and vegetables. Bring to a simmer and reduce until you have a thick, pourable gravy. Remove from the heat and add the kombu, sage, thyme and lemon zest and leave to infuse.

6. Meanwhile, to make the swede purée, put the swede in a pan with the butter. Season with salt and pepper and put on the lid. Place over a medium heat and allow the swede to steam for 30–40 minutes until soft. Transfer into a food processor and blend until smooth.

7. Remove the chicken thighs from the water bath and allow to rest for 20 minutes. Remove the chicken from the bag and put into a frying pan over a medium heat. Cook until the skin is crispy.
8. To serve, spoon some swede purée onto four serving plates, top with a chicken thigh and pour over the gravy.

Guilt-Free Beef Kebabs

Ingredients:

- 10 pcs. cherry tomatoes
- 10 pcs. mushrooms (small)
- 2 tsp. Worcestershire sauce
- ¼ tsp. salt
- 16 oz. beef tenderloin
- 1 green bell pepper cut into squares
- dash of black pepper

Directions:
1. Pre-heat grill
2. Cut the meat into ¾ inch cubes, or about 20 pcs and then sprinkle over with Worcestershire sauce.

3. Using metal skewers, thread the beef, tomatoes, mushrooms, and bell pepper alternately. Sprinkle with pepper.
4. Coat grill with cooking spray and then grill for 10 minutes turning once.
5. Sprinkle with salt before serving.

Blackened Chicken With Avocado

Ingredients:

- 1 tsp. olive oil

- 2 tbsp. cilantro

- 1 finely chopped jalapeno (seeds removed)

- 1 tbsp. freshly squeezed lime juice

- ¼ tsp. salt

- 4 4oz. chicken breast fillet (skin removed)

- 1 avocado (peeled and diced)

- 1 ½ tsp. blackened seasoning

- 1 whole lime cut into 4 wedges

Directions:

1. Sprinkle all sides of chicken with blackened seasoning.
2. Place chicken in a large non-stick skillet pan, drizzled with olive oil, over high heat.
3. Cook the chicken until seared and then reduce to medium heat.
4. Cook again for three minutes or until each side is color brown.
5. In a container, combine avocado, lime juice, jalapeno and salt.
6. Top cooked chicken with avocado mixture and serve with lemon wedges on the side.

Chia Pudding Almond Yogurt Parfait With Warm Cranberries

Ingredients:

- 1 tbsp coconut oil
- 125 g (fresh) Cranberry
- 1 orange (juice)
- 2 tsp maple syrup
- 2 tablespoons almond yogurt
- 2 tablespoons chia seeds
- 1 pinch of vanilla
- 1 pinch of cinnamon
- 250 ml almond milk or other milk plants

Directions:

1. Combine the chia seeds with the cinnamon and vanilla in the almond milk.
2. Allow to simmer for about 20 minutes.
3. The pudding should have a fine creamy consistency and should not be too liquid. (Prepare the chia pudding the night before).
4. In the meantime, place cranberries in a saucepan and simmer at medium temperature with the juice of an orange. Add 2 teaspoons of maple syrup
5. Now add two tablespoons of almond yoghurt to the chia pudding and spread over the warm cranberries.

Spice Porridge With Oranges And Pears

Ingredients:

- 1 pinch of cinnamon
- 1 pinch of turmeric
- 1 pinch of cardamom
- 1 pinch of vanilla
- 5 cloves
- 1 teaspoon coconut oil
- 1 apple
- 1 pear
- 40 g oatmeal
- 1 tbsp flaxseed (not broken)
- 1 tangerine + juice of 1 tangerine

- 200 ml almond milk

- 1 date

- Walnuts to taste

Directions:

1. Cut the date into small pieces and boil with oatmeal and almond milk. Let it swell at medium temperature for 5-7 minutes.
2. Add Linseed, spices and coconut oil to the porridge.
3. Finally, cover with Toppings of fruit and nuts and drizzle with the juice of 1 tangerine.

Totally Awesome Tomato, Cucumber & Over-The-Top Orange Soup

Ingredients:

- 1 cup tomato juice
- 1 small chopped green pepper
- 1 small chopped red pepper, seeds out and core
- 3 large peeled garlic cloves
- 1 orange, juice and zest
- 3/4 cup olive oil
- 1 teaspoon salt
- 1/2 teaspoon pepper
- 7 tomatoes (ripe)

- 1 peeled medium cucumber(no seeds)

- 2 tablespoons apple cider

- 1 small peeled and chopped red onion

- 1 long red chile

- 1 cup cold water

Directions:

1. Take water in a large pot and boil the tomatoes in the boiling water until the skins of the tomatoes get cracked. Remove the tomatoes and clean in cold water then peel off the tomatoes skin and cut into quarter then get rid of the seeds.
2. Next step would be to remove the outer covering of the cucumber and slice in half going lengthwise and eliminate the extra seeds via spoon.

3. Cut all the vegetable process peppers, onion, garlic, tomatoes, chilly, orange zest and cucumber with tomato juice and water in a blender till reasonably soft consistency. Then add vinegar, orange juice, olive oil, pepper, and salt and quickly process until well included but not over-blended so it starts to rise.
4. Depending on the regularity you like, you may add more of tomato juice and/or some water.
5. Serve with the cilantro fillings.

Spicy Chunky Chicken Tangy Tomato Soup

Ingredients:

- 2 cup celery (chopped)
- 30 oz. Of organic chicken broth
- 1 diced sweet onion
- 1 bn. Of finely chopped cilantro
- 4 cloves of minced garlic
- 2 tablespoon tomato (always use paste)
- 1.5 teaspoon chili powder
- 1 teaspoon cumin
- 2 skin removed large chicken breasts and sliced into 1/2 inch strips
- 2 diced jalapenos (de-seeded),

- 1 can of tomatoes (diced)
- 2 cup of ragged carrots
- Pepper (fresh cracked) and sea salt to taste
- Olive oil
- 2 cup water

Directions:
1. Place a drop of oil (olive) and approx. 1/4 cup of chicken broth in a crock pot over med-high heat.
2. Add garlic, jalapeno, onions, pepper and sea salt, cook until easy, adding more of chicken broth as required.
3. Add all the rest of the INGREDIENTS:and sufficient water to seal the top of your crock pot.
4. Cover your crock pot and let the INGREDIENTS:to cook on low heat for about

120 minutes, adjusting the pepper and salt as per the taste.
5. You should be able to cut each piece of chicken easily, once the chicken is cooked properly.
6. Press the ready chicken against the side of the pot using the back of a wooden spoon. Garnish the chicken with fresh cilantro and avocado slices. Enjoy!

Thai Style Tomato Soup

Ingredients:

- 4 tomatoes, heirloom, peeled and chopped finely
- 1 tsp. Of ginger, grated
- Dash of salt and pepper
- 3 cups of vegetable stock
- 1 tsp. Of hot sauce, your favorite brand
- 2 tbsp. Of olive oil
- 1 shallot, medium in size and chopped finely
- 2 cloves of garlic, finely chopped
- 12 inches of grass stalk, lemon and crushed

Directions:

1. Using a large sized soup pot, heat up your olive oil over medium to high heat and then add in your minced garlic and chopped shallot.
2. Sauté these for the next 2 minutes or until fragrant.
3. Then add in the rest of your INGREDIENTS:and allow the soup to cook for the next 20 to 25 minutes.
4. Remove from heat and toss out your lemongrass stalk.
5. Pour your soup into a blender and puree your soup until it reaches the desired consistency that you want.
6. Pour your soup into serving bowls and serve either warm or chilled. Enjoy.

Traditional Mexican Bean Salad

Ingredients:

- 1 avocado, ripe, peeled and sliced finely
- 2 tbsp. Of olive oil
- 2 limes, fresh and juiced
- Dash of salt and pepper for taste
- ½ tsp. Of oregano, dried
- 1 small can of black beans, drained and rinsed
- 1 small can of corn, sweet, drained and rinsed
- 1 cucumber, fresh and sliced thinly
- ½ cup of cilantro, finely chopped
- 1 tomato, ripe, fresh and cut into small cubes

Directions:

1. In a small sized mixing bowl, combine all of your INGREDIENTS:together and toss softly until thoroughly combined.
2. Serve once thoroughly tossed and enjoy.

Avocado Almond Smoothie Bowl

Ingredients:

- Juice of ½ lime, fresh
- ½ cup blueberries, fresh
- 2 tbsp honey
- 1 cup almond milk or almond beverage
- 1 avocado, sliced (reserve ¼ for the topping)
- 2 bananas, frozen & sliced
- 1 cup strawberries, fresh

Directions:

1. Combine the berries together with the bananas, lime juice, avocado, honey & almond drink in a blender. Blend until completely smooth & creamy, preferably on high settings.

2. Pour into bowls & garnish each bowl with the avocado, slivered almonds, and strawberry slices, if desired. Serve immediately

Strawberry Cream Shake

Ingredients:

For strawberry cream shake:

- 1 cup rice-coconut milk, unsweetened (or any plant-based milk)
- 1½ cups strawberries, fresh, remove the green parts
- 3 bananas, frozen & cut into chunks

For chocolate sauce:

- 2 tsp. cocoa powder
- 1 tsp. maple syrup or brown rice syrup or agave syrup
- 2 tsp. water

Directions:

1. In a small pot; add in the cocoa powder, brown rice syrup & water; whisk well & let it cook for a couple of minutes, preferably on low heat settings, then let it cool for a bit, preferably at room temperature.
2. Now, blend strawberries and the rice-coconut milk in a blender, preferably on high settings.
3. Add in the banana chunks; blend again until completely smooth & creamy.

Quinoa Breakfast Cereal

Ingredients:

- Salt to taste //
- 1 tbsp of honey
- 1/2 cup of low-fat milk
- 1 cup of quinoa
- 2 cups of water

Directions:

1. In an enormous pan, add dry quinoa, water, salt, and sugar; mix to consolidate. Heat to the boiling point, lessen warmth to a low-bubble and keep cooking until water has been consumed, roughly 15 minutes.
2. Move to serving bowls, partition warm milk equitably over the oat, and add any fixings wanted.

Directions:

1. To warm tortillas, preheat broiler to 300 degrees.
2. Stack tortillas, envelop by foil, place on a treat sheet, and warm 15 minutes while getting ready fixings.
3. Spot spinach in a food processor and heartbeat until finely hacked, or utilize a blade to dice leaves.
4. In a huge skillet, go to medium-heat, add dark beans and spinach. Warmth until spinach is shriveled, around 3 minutes.
5. Uniformly disperse spinach and bean combination in the wraps (leaving around 2" toward one side for collapsing), add 1/4 cup rice to each wrap, add lettuce, cheddar, salsa, and Greek yogurt equitably overwraps.
6. Crease folds around and under on the finishes.

Chicken Tostadas

Ingredients:

- 1/4 cup cilantro, finely chopped
- 1 tsp cumin
- 1 tsp chili powder
- 3/4 tsp salt
- Lime, juice of
- 15 oz can black beans, drained & rinsed
- 3 cups shredded chicken
- 8 corn tortillas or tostada shells
- 3 medium tomatoes, diced
- 4 medium avocados, diced
- 3 tbsp red onion, finely chopped

- 1/2 cup feta or Cotija cheese

- Cooking spray

Directions:

1. To make tostada shells, line large baking sheet with silicone mat and arrange tortillas in a single layer.
2. Spray with cooking spray and sprinkle with salt on both sides.
3. Bake at 400 degrees for 6 minutes per each side.
4. While tostadas are baking, make easy guacamole salsa by combining tomato, avocado, red onion, cilantro, cumin, chili powder, salt and lime juice. Get other Ingredients: ready.
5. To assemble tostadas, top each shell with guacamole, beans, chicken and cheese.

Instant Pot Stir Fry

Ingredients:

- 2 large garlic cloves, grated
- 2 inch ginger, grated
- 5 tbsp cornstarch
- 12 cups stir fry vegetables, frozen
- 2 lbs (2 large) chicken breasts, frozen
- 1 cup + 4 tbsp water
- 1/3 cup soy sauce (I used Bragg liquid aminos)
- 1/3 cup maple syrup or honey

Directions:

1. In Instant Pot, add 1 cup water, soy sauce, maple syrup, garlic, ginger and place chicken breasts on top.

2. Close the lid, set pressure vent to Sealing and press Pressure Cooking on High for 15 minutes. Display will say ON, Instant Pot will take about 5-7 minutes to come to pressure, you will see a bit of steam coming out from a release valve, then float valve will rise and countdown from 15 minutes will begin.
3. When display says OFF, let Instant Pot bring pressure down on its own for 10 minutes and then turn steam release valve to Venting position until the float valve drops down (if it hasn't dropped down already).
4. Open the lid and using 2 forks, shred chicken breasts.
5. Press Saute on Instant Pot, and in a small bowl whisk together 4 tbsp of water with cornstarch.
6. Add immediately to the pot, stir and cook until thickened.

7. Add frozen vegetables and keep cooking on Sauté until veggies are heated through, stirring every minute.
8. Serve with quinoa or brown rice.

Coffee-Rubbed Steak With Brussels Sprouts Salad

Ingredients:

- 2 teaspoons dijon mustard
- 1 teaspoon honey
- 3 cups shredded brussels sprouts
- 1/3 cup chopped toasted pecans
- 1 ounce blue cheese , crumbled (about 1/4 cup)
- 1 tablespoon ground coffee beans
- 3/4 teaspoon kosher salt , divided
- 3/4 teaspoon black pepper , divided
- 1 pound hanger steak

- 1/4 cup olive oil, divided

- 1 tablespoon apple cider vinegar

Directions:
1. Heat a large cast-iron skillet over medium-high.
2. Stir together coffee, 5/8 teaspoon salt, and 1/2 teaspoon pepper in a small bowl.
3. Sprinkle mixture evenly over steak, pressing gently to adhere.
4. Add 1 tablespoon oil to skillet. Add steak; cook, without moving, until bottom forms a crust, about 3 minutes.
5. Turn steak over; cook until a thermometer inserted in thickest portion registers 120°F, 6 to 7 minutes.
6. Remove from skillet; set aside.
7. Whisk together vinegar, mustard, honey, remaining 3 tablespoons olive oil, remaining

1/4 teaspoon pepper, and remaining 1/8 teaspoon salt in a large bowl.
8. Add Brussels sprouts, pecans, and blue cheese; toss to coat.
9. Slice steak against the grain. Serve with Brussels sprouts salad.

Crispy Salmon Salad With Roasted Butternut Squash

Ingredients:

- 3/4 plus 1/8 tsp. kosher salt , divided
- 1 tablespoon canola oil
- 4 6 4 (6-oz.) skin-on salmon fillets
- 4 cups torn curly kale
- 4 cups baby spinach
- 1/2 cup pomegranate arils
- 2 1/2 cups chopped butternut squash
- 2 1/2 cups sliced red onions
- 1 medium lemon , halved crosswise
- 1/4 cup olive oil

- 1 tablespoon rice vinegar
- 2 teaspoons pure maple syrup
- 1 1/2 teaspoons dijon mustard
- 1/2 teaspoon orange zest
- 3/4 teaspoon black pepper , divided

Directions:
1. Place a baking sheet on rack in upper third of oven; preheat broiler to high.
2. Once hot, carefully remove baking sheet from oven; place squash, onion, and lemon (cut side down) on baking sheet.
3. Broil until charred, 7 to 8 minutes. Let cool; squeeze juice from lemon halves into a small bowl.
4. Whisk together olive oil, vinegar, maple syrup, mustard, orange zest, 1 teaspoon lemon juice,

1/2 teaspoon pepper, and 1/4 teaspoon salt in a medium bowl; set aside.

5. Heat canola oil in a large nonstick skillet over medium-high.
6. Sprinkle salmon flesh with remaining 1/4 teaspoon pepper and remaining 5/8 teaspoon salt.
7. Cook salmon, skin side down, until skin is crisp, 3 to 4 minutes. Flip fillets; cook 2 to 3 minutes.
8. Place kale, spinach, pomegranate arils, squash, and onion in a large bowl.
9. Add vinaigrette; toss to coat. Divide salad and salmon among 4 bowls; spoon 1/2 teaspoon lemon juice over each fillet.

VEGETARIAN RECIPES GOES THUS; White Beans With Roasted Red Pepper And Pesto

Ingredients:

- 1 garlic clove, crushed Beans:
- 1 pound dried Great Northern beans
- 10 cups water, divided
- 1 ½ cups coarsely chopped onion
- 1 tablespoon chopped fresh sage
- 1 tablespoon olive oil
- 2 garlic cloves, crushed
- 1 teaspoon salt
- ¼ teaspoon freshly ground black pepper

- 1 cup chopped bottled roasted red bell peppers
- 2 cups loosely packed basil leaves
- ½ cup (2 ounces) grated fresh Parmesan cheese
- 2 tablespoons pine nuts, toasted
- 2 tablespoons water
- 2 tablespoons extravirgin olive oil
- ¼ teaspoon salt
- ⅛ teaspoon freshly ground black pepper
- 1 tablespoon balsamic vinegar

Directions:

1. To prepare pesto, combine first 8 ingredients in a food processor; process until smooth.

2. To prepare beans, sort and wash the beans. Combine beans
3. To prepare beans, sort and wash the beans.
4. Combine beans quart pressure cooker.
5. Close lid securely; bring to high pressure over high heat.
6. Adjust heat to medium or level needed to maintain high pressure, and cook 3 minutes.
7. Remove from heat; place cooker under cold running water. Remove lid; drain beans.
8. Combine beans, 6 cups water, onion, sage, 1 tablespoon olive oil, and 2 garlic cloves in cooker.
9. Close lid securely; bring to high pressure over high heat.
10. Adjust heat to medium or level needed to maintain high pressure; cook 12 minutes. Remove from heat; place cooker under cold running water.

11. Remove lid; let bean mixture stand for 10 minutes.
12. Drain bean mixture in a colander over a bowl, reserving 1 cup liquid. Return bean mixture and reserved 1 cup liquid to cooker.
13. Add 1 teaspoon salt, 1/4 teaspoon black pepper, bell peppers, and vinegar. Stir well to combine. Top bean mixture with pesto.

Black Lentil And Couscous Salad

Ingredients:

- 1 cup cherry tomatoes, quartered
- ⅓ cup golden raisins
- ⅓ cup finely chopped red onion
- ⅓ cup finely chopped cucumber
- ¼ cup chopped fresh parsley
- 3 tablespoons chopped fresh mint
- 1 teaspoon grated lemon rind
- 3 tablespoons fresh lemon juice
- 2 tablespoons extra-virgin olive oil
- ½ cup dried black lentils
- 5 cups water, divided

- ¾ cup uncooked couscous

- ¾ teaspoon salt, divided

Directions:
1. Rinse lentils with cold water; drain. Place lentils and 4 cups water in a large saucepan; bring to a boil.
2. Reduce heat, and simmer 20 minutes or until tender. Drain and rinse with cold water; drain.
3. Bring remaining 1 cup water to a boil in a medium saucepan; gradually stir in couscous and 1/4 teaspoon salt.
4. Remove from heat; cover and let stand 5 minutes.
5. Fluff with a fork. Combine lentils, couscous, remaining 1/2 teaspoon salt, tomatoes, and remaining ingredients in a large bowl.

Schnitzel With Vegetables

Ingredients:

- 1 tbsp. milk
- 1 tsp. flour
- 1 tbsp. canned horseradish
- 1 tsp. chopped parsley
- 2 veal schnitzel 80g (2.80 oz.)
- 1 tbsp. vegetable oil
- 1 onion
- 1 tsp. butter
- 300g (10.60 oz.) peas
- 100 ml broth
- Salt and pepper

Directions:

1. Chop onions and fry in butter.
2. Add green peas, pour the meat broth and cook within 10 minutes.
3. Mix the milk with the flour and horseradish, add to the centre.
4. Bring everything to a boil; add salt and pepper and sprinkle with parsley.
5. Steak fry with olive oil salt and pepper and serve with peas.

Risotto With Peas

Ingredients:

- 80g (2.80 oz.) rice

- 1 tsp. vegetable oil

- 200ml broth

- 150g (5.30 oz.) green peas

- 1 tbsp. grated cheese

- 1 tsp. butter

- 2 onions cut into small pieces

- 100g (3.5 oz.) cayenne red pepper, finely chopped

- Green onion

- Salt and pepper

Directions:

1. Fry finely chopped onions, bell peppers with rice in hot oil.
2. Pour the broth and boil 15 min.
3. Add peas and grated cheese. Salt and pepper.
4. Sprinkle with finely chopped green onions.

Refrigerator Berry Citrus Breakfast Pudding

Ingredients:

- 1 teaspoon fresh grated ginger

- ¼ cup local honey

- 1 tablespoon pure vanilla extract

- 1 teaspoon cinnamon

- ¾ cup chia seeds

- 1 cup fresh raspberries

- 1 cup fresh blueberries

- 2 cups unsweetened coconut milk

- 1 cup plain Greek yogurt

- 1 lemon, juiced

- 2 teaspoons lemon zest

Directions:

1. In a large bowl, combine the coconut milk, yogurt, and lemon juice. Whisk well.
2. Add the lemon zest, ginger, honey, vanilla extract, cinnamon, and chia seeds. Mix well until evenly combine.
3. Cover and place in the refrigerator overnight.
4. In the morning, stir well, and top with a combination of fresh raspberries and blueberries before serving.

Spicy Morning Breakfast Cocktail

Ingredients:

- 2 cloves garlic, minced and crushed

- 1 tablespoon fresh prepared raw horseradish

- 1 teaspoon Worcestershire sauce

- 2 tablespoons fresh lime juice

- 1 48-ounce bottle tomato juice (plain or spicy)

- 2 teaspoons celery salt

- 1 tablespoon crushed red pepper flakes (adjust to taste)

- 1 teaspoon coarse ground black pepper

- 1 large heirloom tomato, diced

- 2 stalks celery, chopped

- 2 cups fresh spinach, torn
- 1 tablespoon spirulina
- Fresh lime wedges to garnish

Directions:
1. Begin by placing the tomato, celery, spinach, spirulina, and garlic in food processor or blender.
2. Pulse until INGREDIENTS:are chopped and well blended.
3. Add the horseradish, Worcestershire sauce, lime juice, tomato juice, celery salt, crushed red pepper, and black pepper. Blend until smooth.
4. Pour into glasses, over ice if desired.
5. Garnish with fresh lime wedges.

Avocado Toast With Radish Ceviche

Ingredients:

- 2 tbsp olive oil

- large handful fresh dill, finely chopped

- 4 slices sourdough or wholemeal bread

- 2 avocados, peeled and chopped

- 200g pack radishes, sliced very thinly

- 4 limes, juice only

- 2 tsp caster sugar

- 1 small red onion, thinly sliced

- pinch freshly ground black pepper

Directions:

1. Put the radishes in a bowl.

2. Put the lime juice (reserving 2 tablespoons), sugar, red onion, oil and dill in a smaller bowl. Stir, then pour onto the radishes and mix gently. This only needs 10 minutes to infuse.
3. Meanwhile, toast the bread.
4. Mash the avocados with the reserved 2 tablespoons of lime juice to prevent any browning. Spread the toast with the avocados and add a sprinkling of black pepper.
5. Drain the radishes and onions through a colander to remove any excess lime juice, then arrange them on top of the avocado to serve.

Crab With Mango And Avocado Salad

Ingredients:

- 1 red onion, peeled, sliced
- 1 garlic clove, peeled, sliced
- ½ mild red chilli, seeds removed, finely sliced
- 2 sprigs fresh thyme, leaves only
- 1 lime, juice only
- 1-2 tbsp olive oil, or to taste
- pinch salt
- 1kg/2¼lb cooked crab, white meat and claw meat only, chopped (the brown meat can be used in another recipe)
- 1 just-ripe mango, peeled, stone removed, flesh cut into cubes

- 2 avocados, stones and skin removed, flesh cut into cubes

- 2 Little Gem lettuces, leaves separated, washed and patted dry with kitchen paper

Directions:

1. Place the white crabmeat and claw meat into a bowl, add the chopped mango, avocados, red onion, garlic, red chilli, thyme leaves, lime juice and olive oil, then season, to taste, with salt. Mix until well combined.
2. To serve, spoon the crab mixture into the lettuce leaves.
3. Divide the filled lettuce leaves equally among four serving plates.

Grilled Vegetable Wraps With Salsa And Guacamole

Ingredients:

For the salsa

- 8 ripe tomatoes, seeded and diced

- 1 clove of garlic, peeled and crushed

- 1 small onion, peeled and finely chopped

- ¼ fresh green chilli, de-seeded and finely chopped

- 1 tbsp fresh coriander, finely chopped

For the guacamole

- 2 ripe avocados, peeled and stoned

- 1 lime, juice only

- 1 clove of garlic, peeled and crushed

- 1 small onion, peeled and finely chopped
- 3 small tomatoes, seeded and chopped
- ¼ fresh green chilli, de-seeded and finely chopped
- 1 tbsp fresh coriander, finely chopped

For the quesadillas

- 1 courgette, cut into four slices lengthways
- 1 red pepper, seeded and cut into quarters, lengthways
- 1 yellow pepper, seeded and cut into quarters, lengthways
- 1 packet flour tortillas
- coriander leaves, to garnish
- 1 lime, cut into four wedges to garnish

Directions:

1. To make the salsa, mix the tomatoes, garlic, onion, chilli and coriander together and leave for about 30 minutes at room temperature to allow the depth of flavour to develop.
2. To make the guacamole, mash the avocados with the lime juice.
3. Add the garlic, onion, tomato, chilli and coriander and mix thoroughly to combine.
4. To make the quesadillas, heat a chargrill pan over a medium to high heat, add the courgette slices and peppers and grill for 10-15 minutes or until softened and chargrilled in places. Remove the griddled vegetables from the pan and cut into strips.
5. Spread one tablespoon each of guacamole and salsa onto four tortillas.
6. Divide the vegetables between the four tortillas. Wrap them up and return them to the chargrill pan for one minute on each side.

7. Open the quesadilla slightly to serve, garnished with coriander leaves and wedge of lime.

Breakfast: Banana Blueberry Pancakes

Ingredients:

- ¼ cup canola oil
- 1 mashed banana
- 2 tbsp. honey
- 1 cup buttermilk
- ½ cup blueberries
- ½ low-fat milk
- 1 cup oat flour
- 1 cup wheat flour
- 2 eggs
- ½ tsp. baking powder
- 1/2 tsp. baking soda

- 1/4 tsp. salt

Directions:

1. Combine all the dry INGREDIENTS:together in a mixing bowl
2. Take another bowl and combine all the remaining INGREDIENTS:except the blueberries
3. Transfer the wet mixture onto the bowl with the dry Ingredients:.
4. Mix until most of the lumps disappear.
5. Add the blueberries onto the mixture
6. Pour ¼ cup of the mixture onto a hot griddle sprayed with non-stick cooking spray.
7. Cook on both sides until golden, if desired.
8. You can add more berries on the top then drizzle it with maple syrup You can make your own oat flour by simply putting 1 cup of old-fashioned oats into a blender until you get a powdery consistency similar to regular flour.

Chicken With Lemon Garlic Sauce

Ingredients:

- 2 tbsp. Olive oil

- 1 thinly sliced lemon

- ¾ cup low fat milk

- 1 tbsp. Whole wheat flour

- 3 cloves minced garlic

- 3 lbs. Skinless chicken

- 1 tbsp. Freshly squeezed lemon juice

- 1 tbsp. Fresh parsley

- 2 tsp. Fresh thyme

- Salt and pepper to taste

Directions:

1. Sprinkle the chicken with salt and pepper
2. Heat the oil and cook the chicken until browned. While cooking, place the lemon slices on top until the chicken gets cooked through on both sides, then set aside
3. On the same pan, sauté garlic and flour until bubbles appear.
4. Add in the lemon juice, milk, thyme, and parsley. Bring to a boil while continuously whisking. Put it on low heat and simmer for about 5 minutes until it thickens
5. transfer to a serving plate, enjoy

Acai Blackberry Smoothie Bowl

Ingredients:

- 1 teaspoon coarsely ground flaxseed
- 150 ml coconut milk (or milk plants of your choice)
- 1 tsp Coconut oil]
- 1 ripe banana
- 1 ½ tsp Acai powder
- 2 tablespoons oatmeal
- Almonds , sliced banana (fruit of your choice), coconut flakes as toppings

Directions:
1. For the Acai Blackberry Smoothie Bowl, simply pour all the INGREDIENTS:into the blender and mix until a creamy consistency develops.

2. Then garnish the acai smoothie with toppings.

Crazy Carrot, Potatoes & Celery Soup

Ingredients:

- 1 grated and peeled large carrot
- 3 medium peeled white potatoes (small cubes)
- 1/4 thinly sliced white cabbage,
- 1.5 liter vegetable stock
- 2 tablespoons tomato paste
- 1 teaspoon paprika
- 1 teaspoon coriander seeds powder
- 3 tablespoons apple cider
- 1 1/2 teaspoon sea salt
- 2 bay leaves

- 1 teaspoon ghee

- 2 tablespoons of olive oil

- 2/3 black pepper

- A bunch dill (fresh)

- 1 cup of sour cream

- 1 medium peeled brown onion (chop onion finely)

- 3 finely chopped garlic cloves,

- 1 large chopped celery stick,

- 3 medium beets,

Directions:

1. Take a large pot and heat the olive oil and ghee until hot (not at burning point). Fry the celery and chopped onion on a medium heat

for about 5 minutes. Prepare the remaining of the vegetables.
2. Add garlic, also beet root in addition to grated carrots and 1 teaspoon of salt. Sauté and mix together with onion and celery for about 4 minutes.
3. Add coriander seeds powder, tomato paste, black pepper, vinegar and paprika. Mixing through for 1 minute and combine cabbage, potatoes vegetable stock along with bay leaves. Increase the heat to boil.
4. Once the INGREDIENTS:are boiling, decrease the heat and cook for about 20 minutes. Turn off the heat and taste the INGREDIENTS:for salt. You may need to add extra pinch sea salt (depends on the stock you used). The taste of the soup should be little sweet but still spicy with a little sour from the vinegar. The white potatoes should be soft and nice.

5. Before serving, sprinkle 1 1/2 tablespoon of fresh dill (chopped) and let the soup rest, with the lid on, for about 12 minutes.

Crazy Cauliflower & Bacon Soup

Ingredients:

- 1 raw egg
- 1 medium chopped white onion
- 3 chopped garlic cloves
- 3 cup of vegetable stock or perhaps salt reduced chicken
- 2/3 teaspoon of sea salt
- 1/2 teaspoon of grounded black pepper
- 1 medium head of cauliflower (chopped roughly and core out)
- 3/4 cup of bacon (diced)
- 1 tablespoon ghee or 2 tablespoon of olive oil

- coconut oil

Directions:

1. Heat 1 tablespoon of ghee until medium hot in a large pot.
2. Fry the onion for about 5 minutes or until translucent and soft.
3. Boil the stock, cauliflower and garlicup Decrease the heat and cook for 10 approx. minutes.
4. Meanwhile, add the bacon pieces to pan and fry it until crispy.
5. After about 7 to 8 minutes, break the egg into a smaller pan that will fit above the larger pan. Hold the smaller cooking pan close to the heat but not touching the boiling liquid, continue to whisk the egg for about 2 minutes until it gets smooth and frothy (thick yellowish cream). Keep it aside.
6. Take a blender or a food processor and transfer the cauliflower soup to puree until

smooth. Add about 2/3 teaspoon of black pepper and sea salt, process the combination until its smooth.
7. Transfer the egg cream while the blender is still on.
8. Once everything is combined, stop the blender. Taste the soup for salt.
9. Serve with basil or parsley and crispy bacon spread on top.

Chunky Chicken & Vegetable Soup

Ingredients:

- 2 peeled garlic cloves, sliced in two
- 1 teaspoon black pepper
- 8 cups of water (cold)
- 2 teaspoons of salt (sea)
- 1-2 large pans
- 1 chicken (domestic poultry)
- 2 medium peeled white potatoes (sliced into small cubes)
- 2 peeled and washed carrots,
- 2 washed celery sticks,
- 2 green onion(sliced into quarters)

- 3 bay leaves

- some leaves and coriander stems

Directions:

1. Slice the chicken into 4 equally divided pieces. Slice through one side of the breast bone and along the spine on the other side with the help of kitchen scissors. You will get quarters after cutting the thighs from each half. Place the chicken in a big pan and cover it with 8 cups of water. Put it on the stove then increase the hotness to high.
2. Till the time water is boiling prepare the remaining of the Ingredients:. Add the peppercorns, garlic and bay leaves to the stock. Along with the white onion, slice1 of the carrots and 1 of the celery sticks into 3 to 4 pieces and put in to the chicken stock. Save the cilantro for later. The remaining vegetables would be mixed in the second

level. Bring it to boil, then decreasing the heat to low simmer and cover it with a lid. You may skim off the foam but don't worry we are going to drain the liquid. Cook it for about 90 minutes on low heat (it should not boil).
3. You can prepare the remaining vegetables till the time the stock is cooking. Chop and peel the potato, cut the second halves of carrot, celery, and clean the cilantro with water.
4. Smell of the soup should be spread in your home by this stage and you are now prepared for the second level. Remove the pieces of the chicken on to a slicing board and wait for some time. Let the pieces be cool so that we can start working on the meat. Drain the remaining liquid into another pot. Always use freshly sliced veges for crunch.
5. Add carrot, celery, potatoes and salt to the drained stock. Bring the INGREDIENTS:to boil and decrease the heat to low boiling and heat

for about 12 minutes or until the potato is soft and one can easily bite. Remove the skin of the chicken while cooking. Split the meat into thin shreds and come back to the soup, right before serving and then turn the stove off, throw in a handful of diced green onion and coriander leaves some and cover the pan with a lid for a few minutes.

Fresh Spinach And Strawberry Salad

Ingredients:

- 2 tbsp. Of olive oil
- ½ of a lemon, juiced
- Dash of salt and pepper for taste
- 1 tsp. Of vinegar, balsamic
- 1 tsp. Of honey
- 1 pound of spinach, baby and shredded
- ½ cup of strawberries, pureed finely
- 1 cup of strawberries, sliced into halves

Directions:

1. Place your fresh spinach onto a serving plate then place your freshly cut strawberries on top of that and set aside.

2. To make the dressing you will need to combine the rest on your INGREDIENTS:in a small bowl until combined thoroughly.
3. Drizzle your dressing over your salad and serve immediately. Enjoy.

Grilled Balsamic Veggie Salad

Ingredients:

- 1 onion, red in color and sliced finely

- 2 yellow bell pepper, fresh, cored and sliced into quarters

- 2 tbsp. of olive oil

- ¼ cup of vinegar, balsamic

- dash of salt and pepper for taste

- 4 cloves of garlic, chopped finely

- 1 zucchini, fresh and sliced thinly

- 1 eggplant, fresh, peeled and sliced thinly

- 2 tomatoes, ripe and sliced finely

- 1 carrot, fresh and cut lengthwise very finely

Directions:

1. Using a medium sized saucepan, heat it over high heat and place all of your vegetables into it, one by one.
2. Sauté your veggies until they are brown on each side and then remove from heat. Place them into a medium sized mixing bowl.
3. Using a separate bowl mix up your balsamic vinegar, dash of salt and pepper for taste, olive oil and garlic together until evenly combined.
4. Pour your new dressing over your grilled veggies and serve immediately. Enjoy.

Millet With Fruit And Walnuts

Ingredients:

- 4 plums (or fruit of your choice)
- 50 g millet
- 1 cinnamon stick or 1/2 teaspoon cinnamon powder in
- 1 vanilla pod or 1/2 tsp vanilla powder
- 250 ml almond milk
- ½ tsp coconut oil
- 1 tbsp maple syrup
- 1 handful of prunes or fruit at will
- Walnuts

Directions:

1. Wash the plums, remove from them the stones and cut them into small pieces.
2. Mix the millet with the water of the vanilla sauce and add a cinnamon stick with the almond milk.
3. Switch the temperature down and add plums. Allow to simmer for about 5 minutes at low temperature.
4. Finally mix the millet with coconut oil and maple syrup. Serve with walnuts and fruit as desired.

Peanut Butter Green Smoothie

Ingredients:

- 3 Medjool dates, large & pits removed

- 2 large kale leaves, fresh, ribs removed or spinach, fresh

- 2 bananas, frozen

- 2 tbsp. peanut butter or nut butter

- 1 cup non-dairy milk, unsweetened such as organic soy

Directions:

1. Put everything together to a blender & blend until combined, preferably on high settings.
2. Pour the mixture in a tall glass. Serve & enjoy

Golden Turmeric Smoothie

Ingredients:

- ¼ cup peanuts
- 2 tsp turmeric
- ½ cup mango, fresh or frozen
- ¾ cup soy milk or water
- Ice cubes, crushed (approximately ½ cup)
- 2 medjool dates, large, pitted & chopped finely
- ½ cup pineapple, fresh or frozen
- 2 bananas, fresh or frozen

Directions:

1. Put everything together in a blender & blend on high settings until smooth, if required, feel

free to add more of milk or water to get your desired consistency.

Quinoa Salad With Seasonal Vegetables

Ingredients:

- 1 cup of red quinoa, rinsed well
- 2 cups of water, optional vegetable broth
- 2 teaspoons of whole grain mustard
- 3 tablespoons of freshly squeezed lemon juice
- 1 tablespoon of white wine vinegar
- 2 kinds of garlic clove
- 1/4 tsp of red pepper flakes
- Ground black pepper to taste
- Salt to taste
- 1/2 cup of extra-virgin olive oil

Vegetables:

- 1 cucumber, chopped into small chunks
- 1 1/2 cups of whole kernel corn cut from the cob
- 1-pint cherry or grape tomatoes, halved lengthwise
- 1 medium-sized red onion, thinly sliced
- 1/2 cup of chopped Italian parsley

Directions:

1. Get quinoa and 2 cups of water to a bubble in a medium pot over high warmth. Decrease warmth to medium-low, spread, and stew until quinoa is delicate, around 15 minutes. Eliminate pot from the warmth and permit to stand, secured, for 5 minutes. Lighten with a fork. Note: I like to cook the quinoa the day

preceding and refrigerate so that it's as of now cold, and planning time is decreased.

2. Vinaigrette - In a medium bowl, whisk together mustard, lemon juice, white wine vinegar, garlic, red pepper pieces, salt, and pepper. Step by step race in olive oil. Put in a safe spot.
3. In an enormous blending bowl, consolidate cucumber, corn, tomatoes, onion, parsley, and cooled quinoa. Add Vinaigrette to blend and throw delicately. Serve promptly or refrigerate secured until prepared to serve.
4. Simmered Vegetable Directions: for Cool Weather Months: Preheat stove to 400 degrees.
5. While quinoa is cooking, add zucchini and onions to a medium blending bowl, add 2 tablespoons vinaigrette and throw to cover. Spot zucchini and onions on a 13x9x2" non-

stick heating sheet or broiling dish. Spread the vegetables, so they are not contacting.

6. Next, add tomatoes and corn to a similar blending bowl and add 2 tablespoons vinaigrette, throw tenderly to cover, saved.
7. Broil zucchini and onions, revealed, for 20 minutes. Mix vegetables and add tomatoes and corn. Keeping simmering until tomatoes breakdown, around 10 minutes. Eliminate vegetables and put them in a safe spot.
8. In a huge skillet, over medium-low warmth, add quinoa, remaining Vinaigrette, parsley, and extra salt and newly ground dark pepper to taste, stew 2 minutes. Add broiled vegetables to quinoa, throw to consolidate, and cook an extra 2 minutes.

Honey Glazed Salmon With Lemon

Ingredients:

- 1 tablespoon Dijon mustard
- 1 tablespoon freshly squeezed lemon juice
- Sea salt and pepper to taste
- 1 (8 ounces) Wild Alaskan Salmon fillet
- 1 tablespoon honey

Directions:

1. preheat oven to broil.
2. Combine honey, mustard, and lemon juice n a small bowl.
3. Line a rimmed cookie sheet with foil. Spread ¾ honey over salmon, covering both sides. Place salmon on a cookie sheet, drizzle with remaining honey. Place in oven 4-5" from

broiler. Broil 4-5 minutes on each side or until cooked through.

4. If you're a weight trainer, serve over a bed of quinoa or brown rice for an additional 9 grams of protein; otherwise, a side salad is perfect!

Chicken Breast With Tomatoes

Ingredients:

Chicken Breasts:

- 4 large (2-3 lbs) chicken breasts, boneless & skinless
- 1/2 tsp dried oregano
- 1/2 tsp salt
- Ground black pepper, to taste
- Avocado oil

Sauce:

- 4 large (3 lbs) ripe tomatoes, cut into half moon shapes
- 5 garlic cloves, minced
- 1/2 tsp dried oregano

- 1/4 tsp salt

- Ground black pepper, to taste

- Basil or parsley, finely chopped

Directions:

1. Cut chicken breasts into tenders – thin long strips. Sprinkle with 1/2 tsp oregano, 1/2 tsp salt and pepper to taste. Gently toss around the cutting board to coat evenly. Slice tomatoes and chop garlic.
2. Preheat large ceramic non-stick skillet (I used 13") on medium heat and swirl a bit of oil to coat. Add half of chicken and cook for 5 minutes or until golden brown on each side. Transfer to a dish and cook remaining chicken this way, transferring to same dish.
3. Reduce heat to low, add garlic and 1/2 tsp oregano, cook for 1 minute, stirring frequently (add a bit of oil if there was none left from

cooking chicken but there should be). Layer tomatoes on top, sprinkle with 1/4 tsp salt and pepper to taste, turn up the heat to medium, and cook tomatoes for about 5 minutes, gently tossing them around (if tomatoes aren't juicy enough, add a splash of water).

4. When tomatoes have released their juices and turned into fresh tomato sauce, turn off the heat and return chicken back to skillet. Gently tuck it in between tomatoes, sprinkle with fresh basil or parsley, and serve warm with whole wheat spaghetti, quinoa, brown rice or buckwheat.

One Pot Quinoa, Chicken And Broccoli

Ingredients:

Chicken:

- 1/2 tsp all spice (optional but good)
- 1/2 tsp himalayan pink salt
- Ground black pepper, to taste
- 2 lbs boneless & skinless chicken breasts, cut into 1" pieces
- 1 tbsp olive oil, extra virgin*
- 1/2 tsp cumin, ground

Quinoa:

- 1 tsp olive oil, extra virgin
- 1 1/2 cups quinoa, uncooked

- 3 cups boiling water

- 3/4 tsp himalayan pink salt

- 1/2 tsp cumin, ground

- 2 bay leaves

- 1 lb broccoli, chopped

- 2 medium onions, diced

- 3 large garlic cloves, minced

- 1 large carrot, shredded

Directions:

1. Preheat large deep skillet or a dutch oven on medium-high heat. Add Chicken Ingredients: and saute for 10 minutes, stirring occasionally. Drain liquid if necessary and cook until golden brown sides appear. Transfer to a bowl and set aside.

2. Add olive oil, onions, garlic, carrot and cook for 3-5 minutes, stirring occasionally. Add pre-cooked chicken, quinoa, water, remaining salt and cumin, and bay leaves; stir. Bring to a boil, cover, reduce heat to low and cook for 20 minutes.
3. Now it's time to add broccoli. At this point quinoa should be cooked al dente. Add broccoli, stir, cover and cook for 5 more minutes. Serve hot.

Ground Chicken Tacos

Ingredients:

- 1 tbsp organic taco seasoning
- 1 tsp smoked paprika
- 1 cup low sodium tomato sauce
- 1 1/2 cups frozen corn (thawed) or 1 can (drained)
- 1/2 cup cilantro, chopped
- 1 bunch radishes, sliced
- 1 tsp salt
- Organic corn tortillas
- 3 garlic cloves, minced
- 1 large onion, finely chopped

- 2 large bell peppers, finely chopped

- 1 tbsp avocado oil

- 1 lb ground chicken (I used breast)

- Lime, cheese and Greek yogurt, for serving

Directions:

1. Preheat large ceramic non-stick skillet on medium heat and swirl oil to coat.
2. Add garlic and onion, sauté for 2 minutes, stirring occasionally.
3. Add bell pepper and sauté for 7 minutes, stirring occasionally.
4. Add chicken, taco seasoning, smoked paprika and cook for 5 minutes, stirring occasionally and breaking chicken into pieces.
5. Decrease heat to low, add tomato sauce and corn, and cook uncovered for 10 minutes.
6. Add cilantro, radishes and salt; stir.

7. Serve hot over corn tortillas with lime, crumbled feta or shredded Monterey Jack cheese and Greek yogurt.

Eggs Benedict On Greens With Yogurt Hollandaise Sauce

Ingredients:

- 4 large eggs

- 1 cup plain Greek yogurt

- 2 teaspoons lemon juice

- 3 egg yolks

- 1 teaspoon Dijon mustard

- 1 tablespoon fresh dill

- 2 cups endive, chopped

- 2 cups arugula, torn

- 1 cup radish, thinly sliced

- 6 asparagus stalks, sliced very thin lengthwise

- 4 prosciutto slices, sliced into strips
- 1 teaspoon black pepper

Directions:
1. Begin by preparing the salad greens. In a bowl, combine the endive, arugula, radish, and asparagus in a bowl. Toss to combine and distribute evenly among four plates. Top with slices of prosciutto.
2. In the top of a double boiler, combine the Greek yogurt, lemon juice, and egg yolks. Whisk well.
3. Heat over simmering water, whisking frequently, until sauce has thickened, approximately 15 minutes.
4. Meanwhile, add 1½ - 2 inches of water into a saucepan or large skillet. Heat water to a steady simmer.
5. Crack the eggs into ramekins, taking care not to break the yolks. Gently slide the eggs into

the simmering water. Cook until whites are set, approximately 3-4 minutes.
6. Gently lift the eggs out of the water with a slotted spoon and place on the center of the greens.
7. Season the hollandaise sauce with Dijon mustard, dill, and black pepper. Whisk well, and place warm hollandaise sauce over eggs.
8. Serve immediately.

Cinnamon And Maple Sweet Potato Waffles

Ingredients:

- ½ teaspoon salt

- 2 teaspoons cinnamon

- 1 teaspoon ground ginger

- 1 ½ cups sweet potato, cooked and cubed

- 2 eggs, beaten

- 2 teaspoons pure vanilla extract

- ¼ cup pure maple syrup

- 2 teaspoons coconut oil

- ½ cup unsweetened coconut milk

- 1 cup almond flour

- ¼ cup coconut flour

- ½ cup unsweetened shredded coconut
- ½ teaspoon baking soda
- Fresh fruit for garnish, for example, bananas and blueberries

Directions:
1. Begin by preheating the waffle iron.
2. In a large bowl, combine the almond flour, coconut flour, shredded coconut, baking soda, salt, cinnamon, and ginger.
3. In another bowl, combine the sweet potato, eggs, vanilla extract, maple syrup, coconut oil, and coconut milk. Mix well until smooth.
4. In several batches, add the wet INGREDIENTS:to the dry, stirring just until mixed between each addition.
5. Pour the batter into the waffle iron, and cook according to appliance DIRECTIONS:.
6. Serve warm topped with fresh fruit.

Quick Avocado Chocolate Mousse

Ingredients:

- 2 tbsp vanilla extract

- 1 tsp orange extract

- 1 unwaxed orange, finely grated zest only

- 120ml/4fl oz maple syrup

- 10 Medjool dates, finely chopped

- 100ml/3½fl oz milk (or almond milk)

- 2 ripe avocados, halved, stoned and peeled (prepared weight 190g/6½oz)

- 2 ripe bananas, peeled (prepared weight 210g/7½oz)

- 80g/2¾oz good-quality cocoa powder

To finish

- 40g/1½oz good-quality dark chocolate (70% cocoa solids, dairy-free)//
- 50g/1¾oz pecans, toasted and chopped
- 50g/1¾oz macadamia nuts, toasted and chopped
- 1 tsp sea salt flakes

Directions:

1. Put the avocado flesh into a food processor and add the bananas, breaking them into pieces.
2. Add the cocoa powder, vanilla and orange extracts, orange zest, maple syrup, dates and milk. Blend until smooth.
3. Spoon the mousse evenly into glass bowls and grate chocolate over each portion.

4. Sprinkle with the chopped nuts and sea salt flakes to serve.

www.ingramcontent.com/pod-product-compliance
Lightning Source LLC
Chambersburg PA
CBHW071457080526
44587CB00014B/2131